Tuberculosis – India is fighting for elimination

Weaker private sector in managing TB: Drug Resistant TB - a big challenge

Sanjay Suryawanshi

ELIVA PRESS

Sanjay Suryawanshi

Tuberculosis (TB) is a major contagious infection that usually attacks lungs and it spreads to other parts of body like brain, spine etc. It is caused by the bacteria called M Tuberculosis. In many low-income, middle-income countries, TB continues to be a major cause of morbidity & mortality, and drug-resistant TB is a major concern in many settings.

India is the highest TB burden country in the world having an estimated incidence of 26.9 lakh cases in 2019 (WHO) with high Drug Resistant TB as well and HIV TB. Approximately 50 % or even more TB patients are accountable to private sector leading lower TB notification. India has now developed the ability to achieve complete surveillance coverage including mandatory private sector notification, putting efforts at all levels of program management to ensure complete and adequate diagnostics, treatment and preventive services.

TB infection does not necessarily mean someone get the disease but there is a probability based on poor immune status. There are two variants commonly observed, latent TB where TB bacteria present in body but no symptoms as the immunity is stronger one and active TB means bacteria multiply and one can become sick and further transmit the disease. 90 % of active TB cases are form latent TB infection.

When someone coughs, sneezes, talks, laughs, or sings etc, they release tiny droplets that contain the germs and if someone breathe in these germs, can get it. Major symptoms seen are cough, fever, chest pain, coughing of blood, weight loss etc

It is always risky for any one if a friend, co-worker, or family member has active TB, travelled in any risk area or associated with risk groups like HIV, DM, people living with congregate settings (jail, prisons) or health worker in general or high TB settings (TB wards).

Today with best drugs available TB is completely curable, but it takes longer time (6-9 months in DSTB, 20 months in DRTB). Even then it is mandatory to stop transmission in community by early diagnosis and prompt treatment and adopting simplest measures cough etiquettes, hand washing, health education etc. In present era treatment of LTBI is important part of TB elimination and on top of TB elimination agenda.

Published: Eliva Press SRL
Address: MD-2060, bd.Cuza-Voda, 1/4, of. 21 Chişinău, Republica
Moldova
Email: info@elivapress.com
Website: www.elivapress.com

ISBN: 978-1-63648-005-3

Contents

High unfavourable outcomes among patients with MDR-TB on standard 24 month regimen in Maharashtra, India

ABSTRACT

Setting: Patients with MDR-TB registered for treatment (2011-12 cohort) using the standard 24 month regimen, Programmatic Management of Drug-resistant TB (PMDT) under Revised National TB Control Programme, Maharashtra, India
Objectives: To assess the treatment outcomes; and the timing and risk factors for unfavourable treatment outcomes with focus on death and loss to follow up.
Method: Retrospective cohort study involving review of PMDT records. Treatment outcomes were reported on 31 Dec 2014.
Results: Of 4024 patients, after excluding those with missing treatment outcomes (n=375) and those still on treatment (n=239), 3410 patients were included. Treatment success was seen in 1168 (34%) patients. Unfavourable outcomes were seen in 2242 (66%): 857 (24%) died; and 768 (21%) were loss to follow up. Half of loss to follow up occurred within three months and more than four-fifth of deaths occurred after six months of treatment. HIV, underweight, age ≥15 years, male sex and pulmonary TB were the risk factors for death or loss to follow up or unfavourable treatment outcomes.
Conclusion: The study found poor treatment outcomes in patients with MDR-TB registered for treatment in Maharashtra, India. Interventions are required to address high loss to follow up and deaths.

INTRODUCTION

Globally, multi drug resistant tuberculosis (MDR-TB) poses a major threat to the ongoing efforts for tuberculosis control. In 2015, globally there were 580,000 estimated new cases of MDR-TB and Rifampicin resistant TB (RR-TB); among them 125,000 (20%) were enrolled. The MDR-TB treatment success rate was 52% for the 2013 cohort.[1]

India, China and the Russian Federation accounted for 45% of all estimated MDR/RR-TB cases (henceforth to be called as MDR-TB). India, one of the countries with high burden of TB, has an estimated 79,000 MDR-TB cases among notified pulmonary TB cases. [1]

The Revised National TB Control Programme (RNTCP) of India has made substantial progress to diagnose and treat MDR-TB cases through its programmatic management of MDR-TB (PMDT) since 2007. The PMDT services witnessed accelerated scale up to all districts in India by March 2013. The laboratory confirmed patients with MDR-TB are initiated on standardized regimen for DR-TB that extends from 24 to 27 months. [2] The recent available MDR-TB treatment success rate for the 2013 cohort is 46%. [1,3]

Maharashtra state is the second largest province situated in the western part of India and has a population of 118 million[4] with 79 district level reporting units under RNTCP,[5] with headquarters at Mumbai, the megacity with the highest burden of MDR-TB in India.[6]

In this paper we report the treatment outcomes; and the timing and risk factors for unfavourable treatment outcomes with focus on death and loss to follow up among a large cohort of patients with MDR-TB registered for treatment using the standard 24 month regimen under PMDT between 2011 and 2012 in the Maharashtra, India.

METHODS

Study design and population

The study was a retrospective cohort study involving review of PMDT records of patients with MDR-TB registered for treatment between January 2011 and December 2012, at all DR-TB centres (n=11) across Maharashtra, India..

Study setting

Diagnosis of MDR-TB was done through ten culture and drug susceptibility testing (C-DST) laboratories certified under RNTCP for various WHO endorsed diagnostics (Xpert MTB-Rif, LPA, Liquid and Solid culture-DST) for majority of patients and Xpert MTB-Rif standalone laboratories (n=4) initiated in 2012. Follow up cultures were done through liquid or solid cultures. The sputum samples from the presumptive MDR-TB cases and laboratory confirmed patients with MDR-TB were transported from collection centers of all districts to the linked laboratories either by courier agency or programme personnel in properly packed falcon tubes maintained in cold chain under bio-safety environment. Since 2015, five laboratories have also advanced to offer baseline second line DST in liquid culture.

All laboratory confirmed patients with MDR=TB or Rifampicin Resistant TB (RR-TB) underwent pre-treatment evaluation and were initiated on standardized treatment regimen at 11 DR-TB centers suitably upgraded with airborne infection control measures and managed by a team of trained clinical specialists. After an initial short period of hospitalization, they were shifted to their domicile, to continue their rest of standard DR-TB treatment on ambulatory basis. The duration of DR-TB treatment was for 24-27 months that consisted of at least six months and a maximum of nine months of intensive phase [Kanamycin, Levofloxacin, Ethionamide, Pyrazinamide, Ethambutol and Cycloserine] and 18 months of continuation phase [Levofloxacin, Ethionamide, Ethambutol and Cycloserine]. These patients were monitored by sputum culture examination at 3,4,5,6 months during intensive phase and quarterly in continuation phase at 7, 9,12,15,18,21 and 24 month.[2] Patients were reviewed after six months and treatment was shifted to continuation phase if the recent culture result available at the end of six months of treatment was culture negative. If the recent culture was positive at the end of six months of treatment (4 month with solid culture / 5 month with liquid culture in some cases), the intensive phase was extended by one month; and further extension beyond one month was based on the culture result of 5, 6 and 7 month as these culture results became available. The IP could be extended for maximum of three months based on positive culture result at 4, 5, 6, 7 month.

Variables and source of data

Data collection from PMDT treatment registers maintained at all DR-TB centres of Maharashtra was done between April and June 2015. The variables collected in the data collection form included registration number, DR-TB centre, date of registration, age, sex, weight bands, HIV status, site of TB, previous TB category, treatment outcome and date of outcome. Time between diagnosis and treatment registration was derived in days from the respective dates. Treatment outcomes were defined as per PMDT guidelines and have been defined in **Box below**.[2] 'Cured' and 'treatment completed' were classified as favourable treatment outcomes (treatment success); and rest were classified as unfavourable treatment outcomes. Treatment outcomes were reported on 31 Dec 2014.

Box : MDR-TB treatment outcomes according to Programmatic Management of DR-TB guidelines, Revised National TB Control Programme, India [2]

Cure: *A patient who has completed treatment and has been consistently culture negative (with at least 5 consecutive negative results in the last 12 to 15 months). If one follow-up positive culture is reported during the last three quarters, patient will still be considered cured provided this positive culture is followed by at least 3 consecutive negative cultures, taken at least 30 days apart, provided that there is clinical evidence of improvement.*

Treatment completed: *A patient who has completed treatment according to guidelines but does not meet the definition for cure or treatment failure due to lack of bacteriological results.*

Treatment failure: *Treatment will be considered to have failed if two or more of the five cultures recorded in the final 12-15 months are positive, or if any of the final three cultures are positive.*

Death: *A patient who dies for any reason during the course of M/XDR-TB treatment ? Treatment default: A patient whose treatment was interrupted for two or more consecutive months for any reasons.*

Transfer out: *A patient who has been transferred to another reporting unit (DR-TB Centre in this case) and for whom the treatment outcome is not known. Till the time the PMDT services are available across the country, the M/XDR TB patients can be transferred out only to those districts, within or outside the state, where these services are available. If a patient moves from one district to another, both of which are covered by the same DR-TB Centre, transfer out will not be required.*

Treatment stopped due to adverse drug reactions: *A patient who develops severe adverse reactions and could not continue the M/XDR-TB treatment in spite of the management of the adverse reactions as per the defined protocols and decision has been taken by the DR-TB Centre committee to stop treatment*

Treatment stopped due to other reasons: *A patient who could not continue the M/XDR-TB treatment for any other medical reason (than adverse drug reactions), and a decision has been taken by the DR-TB Centre committee to stop treatment.*

Switched to Regimen for XDR TB: *A MDR-TB patient who is found to have XDR-TB by an RNTCP certified C-DST laboratory, who subsequently switched to a regimen for XDR TB treatment initiated.*

Still on treatment: *An M/XDR-TB patient who, for any reason, is still receiving their treatment at the time of the submission of the Treatment Outcome Report*

Data management and analysis

Data were collected and entered by the statistical assistant of all DR-TB centres with support from district DR-TB supervisors under the supervision of District TB Officer or medical officer in-charge. All the concerned staff were a priori trained in data entry. The data from each DR-TB site were double entered, validated, appended and analysed using EpiData (version 3.1 for entry and validation; version 2.2.2.183 for merging and analysis, EpiData Association, Odense, Denmark).

Key analytic outputs were frequency and proportion of patients with unfavourable treatment outcome. Death and loss to follow up were stratified by phase of treatment (<3 months, 3-6 months, 6-24 months and end of treatment). Risk factors were identified separately for unfavourable treatment outcomes, deaths and loss to follow up. Unadjusted relative risks and 0.95 CI were used to summarize and infer the association after removing the records with missing variable of interest. We decided against performing a regression analysis because of significant number of missing data for key exposure variables.

Ethics

Ethics approval to conduct the study was obtained from Ethics Advisory Group (EAG) of International Union against Tuberculosis and Lung Disease (The Union), Paris and Ethics Committee of National Tuberculosis Institute, Bengaluru, India. Waiver of informed consent was requested and sought as this study involved retrospective record review of routinely collected program data. Permission from the tuberculosis state programme manager of Maharashtra was obtained for the conduct of the study.

RESULTS

The treatment outcomes and the timing of the treatment outcomes have been shown in **Figure below**.

Of 4024 patients, treatment outcomes were not recorded for 375 and treatment was still going on for 239. A total of 3410 patients were included in the final analysis. Among patients with dates available (n=3104), median (IQR) time in days to register after diagnosis was 41 (25, 71) with 6% patients (183/3104) getting registered within 14 days.

Treatment success was seen in 1168 (34%) patients and rest had unfavourable treatment outcomes. A total of 828 (23%) were declared cured; 340 (9%) completed treatment, 857 (24%) died during treatment; 768 (21%) were loss to follow up; 98 (3%) failed treatment; 190 (5%) were switched to Category V; treatment was stopped due to adverse drug reaction for 3 (<1%) and due to other causes in 29 (<1%); and 297 (8%) were not evaluated after transfer out. **Table I** summarises the timing of death and loss to follow up during treatment. Among 768 patients with loss to follow, 379 (49%) occurred within first three months. Among 857 patient who died, 722 (84%) occurred in the continuation phase.

Figure. Flow chart describing the timing of treatment outcomes of Patients with MDR-TB registered for treatment in Maharashtra,2011-12

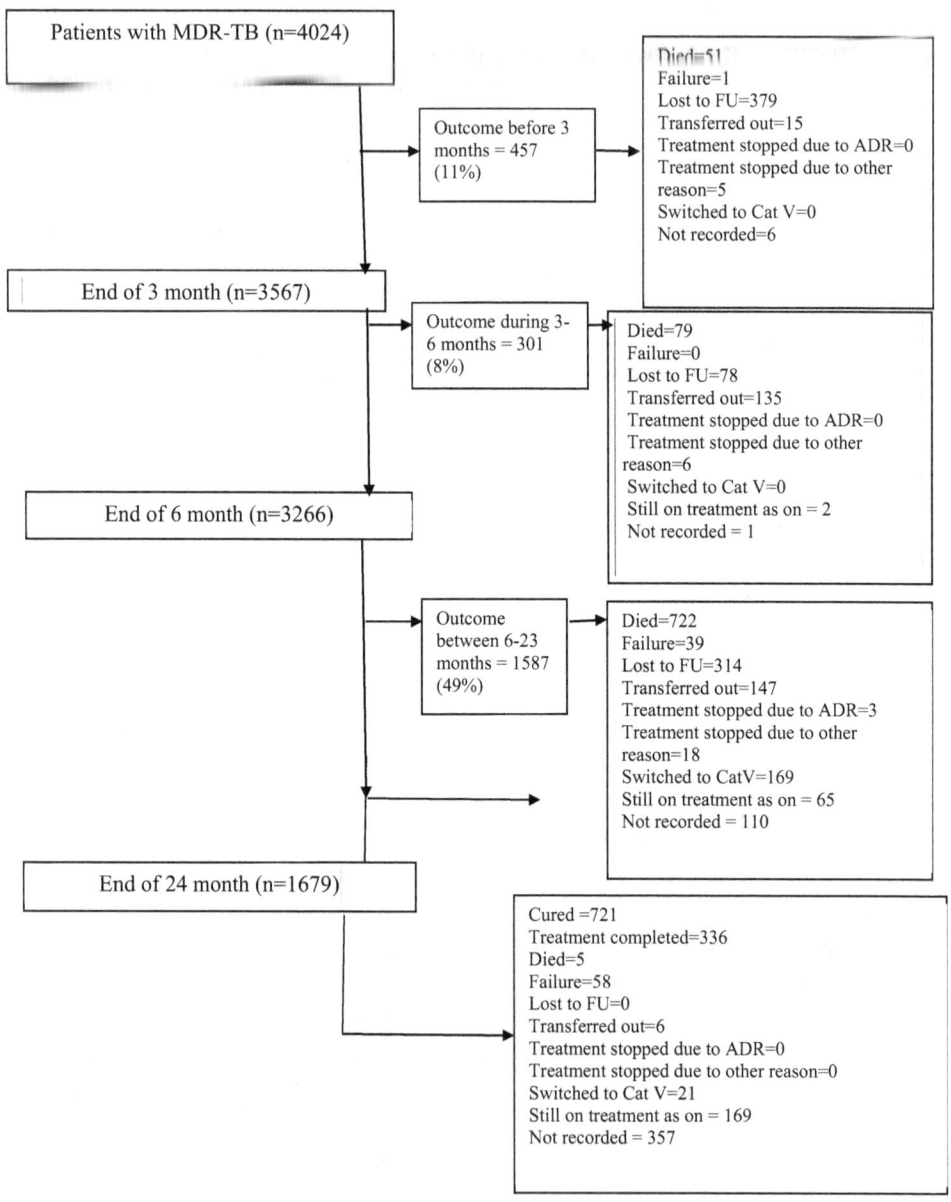

Patients with MDR-TB (n=4024)

Outcome before 3 months = 457 (11%)

Died=51
Failure=1
Lost to FU=379
Transferred out=15
Treatment stopped due to ADR=0
Treatment stopped due to other reason=5
Switched to Cat V=0
Not recorded=6

End of 3 month (n=3567)

Outcome during 3-6 months = 301 (8%)

Died=79
Failure=0
Lost to FU=78
Transferred out=135
Treatment stopped due to ADR=0
Treatment stopped due to other reason=6
Switched to Cat V=0
Still on treatment as on = 2
Not recorded = 1

End of 6 month (n=3266)

Outcome between 6-23 months = 1587 (49%)

Died=722
Failure=39
Lost to FU=314
Transferred out=147
Treatment stopped due to ADR=3
Treatment stopped due to other reason=18
Switched to CatV=169
Still on treatment as on = 65
Not recorded = 110

End of 24 month (n=1679)

Cured =721
Treatment completed=336
Died=5
Failure=58
Lost to FU=0
Transferred out=6
Treatment stopped due to ADR=0
Treatment stopped due to other reason=0
Switched to Cat V=21
Still on treatment as on = 169
Not recorded = 357

Table I. Timing of death and loss to follow up among Patients with MDR-TB registered for treatment under RNTCP between 2011-12, Maharashtra, India (n=3410)

Phase of treatment	Death N (%)	Loss to follow up N (%)
Total	**857 (100)**	**768 (100)**
<3 months	51 (6)	379 (49)
3- 6 months	79 (9)	78 (10)
6-24 months	722 (84)	311 (40)
End of treatment	5 (1)	0 (0)

Tables II-IV show factors associated with unfavourable treatment outcome, death and loss to follow up respectively. Factors associated with unfavourable outcome were all age groups ≥15 years (when compared to <15 years); male sex (when compared to female sex); pulmonary TB (when compared to extra pulmonary – non lymph node involvement); and weight bands 16-25 kg and 26-45 kg (when compared to >70 kg). Factors associated with death were: weight bands 16-25 kg and 26-45 kg (when compared to 46-70 kg); pulmonary TB (when compared to extra pulmonary – non lymph node involvement); and those with HIV co-infection. Treatment initiation within 14 days was associated with death. Male sex was associated with loss to follow up when compared to female sex and weight band 16-25 kg was associated with reduced risk for loss to follow up when compared to >70 kg.

Table II. Risk factors associated with unfavourable outcomes among Patients with MDR-TB, registered for treatment under RNTCP between 2011-12, Maharashtra, India (n=3410)

Variable^		Total	Unfavourable outcomes		RR (0.95 CI)	
		N	n	%		
Total		**3410**	**2242**	**66**	-	
Age in years						
	<15	78	39	50	Ref	
	15-44	2695	1746	65	1.3(1.0,1.6)*	
	45-64	579	418	72	1.4(1.2,1.8)*	
	>/=65	58	39	67	1.3(1.0,1.8)*	
Sex						
	Female	1401	858	61	Ref	
	Male	2009	1384	69	1.1(1.1,1.2)*	
TB site						
	PTB	3323	2211	67	2.3(1.6,3.5)*	
	EPTB-LN	24	11	46	1.6(0.9,2.9)	
	EPTB-Others	59	17	29	Ref	
	Missing	4	-	-	-	
Previous TB category						
	New	496	310	63	Ref	
	Retreatment	2002	1318	66	1.1(0.9,1.1)	
	Missing	912	-	-	-	
HIV status						
	Positive	138	82	59	0.9(0.8,1.1)	
	Negative	2457	1573	64	Ref	
	Unknown	116	71	61	0.96(0.8,1.1)	
	Missing	699	-	-	-	
Time between diagnosis and registration						
	<15 days	183	131	672	Ref	
	>/=15 days	2921	1903	65	0.9 (0.8,1.0)	
	Missing	306	-	-	-	

Weight in kg					
	<16	5	1	20	-
	16-25	127	95	75	1.8(1.2,2.7)*
	26-45	2229	1533	69	1.6(1.1,2.5)*
	46-70	1012	597	59	1.4(0.9,2.1)
	>70	31	13	42	Ref
	Missing	6	-	-	-

MDR-TB= Multidrug resistant TB; RNTCP=Revised national tuberculosis control programme; RR= Relative risk; CI=Confidence interval;, HIV=Human Immunodeficiency Virus; EPTB=Extra pulmonary TB, LN=Lymph node; PTB=Pulmonary TB; * statistically significant; ^Row percentages; missing variables have been mentioned but not included in the unadjusted analysis

Table III. Risk factors associated with death among Patients with MDR-TB, registered For treatment under RNTCP between 2011-12, Maharashtra, India (n=3410)

Variable		Total	Death		RR (0.95 CI)
		N	n	%	
Total		**3410**	**857**	**25**	-
Age in years					
	<15	78	15	19	Ref
	15-44	2695	654	24	1.3(0.8,2.0)
	45-64	579	171	30	1.5(0.96,2.5)
	>/=65	58	17	29	1.5(0.8,2.8)
Sex					
	Female	1401	346	25	Ref
	Male	2009	511	25	1.03(0.9,1.2)
TB site					
	PTB	3323	850	26	3.0(1.3,7.0)*
	EPTB-LN	24	0	0	-
	EPTB-	59	5	9	Ref
	Others	4	-	-	-
	Missing				
Previous TB category					
	New	496	115	23	Ref
	Retreatment	2002	532	27	1.2(0.96,1.4)
	Missing	912	-	-	-
HIV status					
	Positive	138	52	38	1.5(1.2,1.9)*
	Negative	2457	606	25	Ref
	Unknown	116	30	26	1.1(0.8,1.4)
	Missing	699	-	-	-
Time between diagnosis and registration					
	<15 days	183	59	32	Ref
	>/=15 days	2921	713	24	0.8 (0.6, 0.9)*
	Missing	306	-	-	-

Weight in kg					
	<16	5	1	20	-
	16-25	127	61	48	3.9(3.1,5.0)*
	26-45	2229	668	30	2.5(2.1,2.9)*
	46-70	1012	124	12	Ref
	>70	31	1	3	-
	Missing	6	-	-	-

*MDR-TB= Multidrug resistant TB; RNTCP=Revised national tuberculosis control programme; RR= Relative risk; CI=Confidence interval;, HIV=Human Immunodeficiency Virus; EPTB=Extra pulmonary TB, LN=Lymph node; PTB=Pulmonary TB; * statistically significant; ^Row percentages; missing variables have been mentioned but not included in the unadjusted analysis*

Table IV. Risk factors associated with loss to follow up among Patients with MDR-TB, registered for treatment under RNTCP between 2011-12, Maharashtra, India (n=3410)					
Variable		**Total**	**Loss to follow up**		**RR (0.95 CI)**
		N	n	%	
Total		**3410**	**768**	**23**	-
Age in years					
	<15	78	10	13	Ref
	15-44	2695	585	22	1.7(0.95, 3.0)
	45-64	579	158	27	2.0 (0.98, 4.2)
	>/=65	58	15	26	
Sex					
	Female	1401	221	16	Ref
	Male	2009	547	27	1.7 (1.5, 2.0)*
TB site					
	PTB	3323	752	23	1.3 (0.8, 2.4)
	EPTB-LN	24	5	21	1.2 (0.5, 3.2)
	EPTB-Others	59	10	17	Ref
	Missing	4	-	-	-
Previous TB category					
	New	496	105	21	Ref
	Retreatment	2002	426	21	1.0 (0.8,1.2)
	Missing	912	-	-	-
HIV status					
	Positive	138	21	15	0.7 (0.5, 1.1)
	Negative	2457	517	21	Ref
	Unknown	116	31	27	1.3(0.9, 1.7)
	Missing	699	-	-	-
Time between diagnosis and registration					
	<15 days	183	41	22	Ref
	>/=15 days	2921	668	23	1.0 (0.7, 1.4)
	Missing	5	-	-	-

Weight in kg					
	<16	5	0	0	-
	16-25	127	8	6	0.3 (0.1, 0.7)*
	26-45	2229	452	20	0.9 (0.5, 1.7)
	46-70	1012	301	30	1.3 (0.7, 2.6)
	>70	31	7	23	Ref
	Missing	6	-	-	-

MDR-TB= Multidrug resistant TB; RNTCP=Revised national tuberculosis control programme; RR= Relative risk; CI=Confidence interval;, HIV=Human Immunodeficiency Virus; EPTB=Extra pulmonary TB, LN=Lymph node; PTB=Pulmonary TB; * statistically significant; ^Row percentages; missing variables have been mentioned but not included in the unadjusted analysis

DISCUSSION

This large cohort of patients with MDR-TB from Maharashtra had long turnaround time to register after diagnosis and high proportion of unfavourable treatment outcomes. More than two-thirds of unfavourable outcomes were due to death and loss to follow up. Significant numbers of patients were lost to follow up in the first three months of treatment. Risk factors associated with unfavourable treatment outcomes were identified.

The study had several strengths. This was a very large cohort that included all patients registered for DR-TB treatment over a period of two years in one of the largest states of India. Since we studied the entire population of patients without any sampling, the results are likely to be representative and reflect the ground reality. Double data entry and validation ensured quality assured and robust data. This operational research was conducted without additional funding within existing programme settings. We followed STROBE guidelines to report the findings of the study. [7]

There are inherent limitations of a record review study, but, records in RNTCP are monitored and supervised which includes periodic data validation. Despite this, the key limitation was a significant number of missing records for exposure variables (Table 1-3) and treatment outcomes (n=375). This prevented us from utilizing entire cohort in our analysis and from performing regression analysis for adjusted associations. We used date of registration as date of treatment initiation was not uniformly available.

Overall the treatment success rate of 34% was very low compared to the WHO reported global estimate of 52% and the national figure of 46% for India. [1,3] This is even lower when compared to WHO 2015 target of at least 75% treatment success of MDR-TB.[8] Similar low treatment success was reported from Tamil Nadu, a state in south India, with treatment success in the range of 30-41%.[9]

Six out of ten loss to follow up happened in intensive phase of treatment: majority happening within the first three months itself. Considering high proportions of patients were lost to follow up early during treatment, there is a need for counselling for DR-TB treatment at least in the intensive phase of treatment. Eight out of ten deaths happened in continuous phase of treatment

The risk factors identified for unfavourable treatment outcome in the study like low weight band, HIV and male sex, among many others, require special attention within the programme. Poor treatment outcomes among a cohort of HIV co-infected patients have been described from Mumbai, India and Johannesburg, South Africa. [10,11] Malnutrition has also been associated with unfavourable treatment outcomes. [12,13] Timely initiation of ART or continuation on ART if receiving already through effective TB-HIV linkage, nutritional supplementation for patients in low weight band and treatment adherence support has helped in reducing deaths and loss to follow up; ensuring a treatment success of 79%. [14]

Only one in 16 patients was initiated on treatment within 14 days and it was a risk factor for death. We assume that many of these patients would have been sick and contributed to higher risk of death. As mentioned previously, adjusted analysis was not possible to determine the independent effect due to missing data. Weight band 16-25 kg was associated with reduced risk for loss to follow up. We can explain this as patients with low baseline weight would have been on close follow up. Death was more common than loss to follow up among this weight band.

In our study, second line DST was done among MDR-TB if they satisfied the presumptive Extensively Drug Resistant TB (XDR-TB) criteria.[2] Following this, 190 (5.2%) were identified as XDR and switched to XDR-TB regimen. We assume many patients with undetected XDR-TB either died or were lost to follow up as second line DST was not done at baseline. Considering the high number of unfavourable outcomes, from 2015 onwards, all patients with MDR-TB in Maharashtra underwent second line DST at baseline. As a result 899 patients with XDR-TB were registered on treatment in Maharashtra alone: this was 42% (899 / 2130) of the total XDR detected in the country. According to annual report of RNTCP in 2016, baseline second line DST has been introduced as a policy for all patients with MDR-TB. [3] Future research is required to document its implementation and impact on MDR-TB treatment outcomes.

In May 2016, WHO has recommended a standardized 9-12 months regimen for all patients (excluding pregnant women) with pulmonary MDR-TB that is not resistant to second line drugs. Clofazimine and linezolid are now recommended as core second- line medicines in the MDR-TB regimen, whereas Bedaquiline and Delamanid have been included as specific subgroup of add-on agents.[1,15] At least 23 countries in Asia and Africa have introduced shorter regimens for treatment of MDR-TB and have documented high treatment success rates (87–90%) under operational research conditions.[1] In India, Bedaquiline has been given approval for use for first six months of treatment along with the background 24 month regimen under conditional access through the RNTCP PMDT programme in six referral sites. This is to assess the safety profile of the drug among Indian population. [3]

Policy implications: There are many policy implications of this study. First, there is a need to improve routine data recording at the DR-TB centres in Maharashtra. Second, the programme needs to address the long delay in registering the patients. Third, the way forward for the RNTCP PMDT in Maharashtra, India is to reduce deaths during treatment by addressing high risk groups like HIV co-infection, malnutrition through better implementation of TB-HIV collaborative services and nutritional supplementation respectively; reduce loss to follow up by providing counselling services for patients with MDR-TB, at least during the intensive phase; and ensure high coverage of baseline DST among MDR-TB patients to detect underlying FQ resistance or XDR-TB. International Union Against Tuberculosis and Lung Disease (The Union) has supported provision of MDR-TB counsellors in the state; the effect of the same on treatment outcomes needs to be evaluated in the future. Considering the poor outcomes of the current 24 months in the state as well as the country as a whole, the programme may consider implementing the WHO recommended shorter MDR-TB regimen which has found high success rates in other operational settings around the world. [1,15]

CONCLUSION

In conclusion, the study found poor treatment outcomes in patients with MDR-TB registered for treatment in Maharashtra, India. Interventions are required to address high loss to follow up and deaths for the program to achieve the target of ending the epidemic of TB by 2030 and 2035 in line with the recently released Sustainable Development Goals and end TB strategy respectively. [16,17]

Acknowledgements

We would like to acknowledge the support from the RNTCP programme staff who helped us in performing the record review.

Data availability statement

The database along with codebook and the programme used for analysis may be made available upon request to corresponding author.

Role of Investigators

SLS: Principal Investigator; **HDS:** corresponding author; **SLS, SBN, HDS**: conception / design of the protocol; **SLS, SBN:** development of data collection tool; **SLS, SBN:** acquisition of data and data entry; **HDS, SAN, MP:** data analysis / interpretation; **HDS:** preparing first draft; **all authors** critically reviewed the paper and gave approval for the final version to be published

Funding

The study was conducted as a part of the 'TB Operations Research Training Project' aimed to build operational research capacity within the Government of India's RNTCP. This training project was conceived and implemented jointly by Central TB Division (Directorate General of Health Services, Ministry of Health and Family Welfare, Government of India), the National TB Institute (Directorate General of Health Services, Ministry of Health and Family Welfare, Government of India Bangalore, India), World Health Organization (India Country Office), The International Union Against Tuberculosis and Lung Diseases (The Union, South-East Asia Regional Office, New Delhi, India) and U.S. Centers for Disease Control and Prevention (Division of TB Elimination, Atlanta, USA). We thank the Department for International Development (DFD), UK, for funding the Global Operational Research Fellowship Programme at the International Union Against Tuberculosis and Lung Disease (The Union), Paris, France in which Hemant Deepak Shewade works as an operational research fellow.

REFERENCES

1. World Health Organization (WHO). Global Tuberculosis Report 2016. Geneva, Switzerland; 2016.
2. Revised National Tuberculosis Control Programme. Guidelines on Programmatic Management of Drug Resistant TB (PMDT) in India. New Delhi India; 2012.
3. Revised National Tuberculosis Control Programme. TB India 2016.

Annual status report. New Delhi India; 2016.

4. Government of India. Ministry of Home Affairs. Office of Registrar General and Census Commissioner. Census of India [Internet]. 2011 [cited 2016 May 27]. Available from: http://www.censusindia.gov.in/2011-common/ccnsus_2011.html

5. Revised National Tuberculosis Control Porgramme (RNTCP). TB India 2013. Annual Status Report. New Delhi; 2013.

6. Mistry N, Tolani M, Osrin D. Drug-resistant tuberculosis in Mumbai, India: An agenda for operations research. Operations Research for Health Care. 2012;1:45–53.

7. von Elm E, Altman DG, Egger M, Pocock SJ, Gøtzsche PC, Vandenbroucke JP. The Strengthening the Reporting of Observational Studies in Epidemiology (STROBE) Statement: Guidelines for reporting observational studies. The Lancet. 2007;370:1453–1457.

8. World Health Organization (WHO). The Global Plan to Stop TB: 2011–2015. Geneva, Switzerland; 2010.

9. Nair D, Navneethapandian PD, Tripathy JP, et al. Impact of rapid molecular diagnostic tests on time to treatment initiation and outcomes in patients with multidrug-resistant tuberculosis, Tamil Nadu, India. Transactions of the Royal Society of Tropical Medicine and Hygiene. 2016;

10. Isaakidis P, Paryani R, Khan S, et al. Poor outcomes in a cohort of HIV-infected adolescents undergoing treatment for multidrug-resistant tuberculosis in Mumbai, India. PloS one. 2013;8:e68869.

11. Umanah T, Ncayiyana J, Padanilam X, Nyasulu PS. Treatment outcomes in multidrug resistant tuberculosis-human immunodeficiency virus Co-infected patients on anti-retroviral therapy at Sizwe Tropical Disease Hospital Johannesburg, South Africa. BMC infectious diseases. 2015;15:478.

12. Hicks RM, Padayatchi N, Shah NS, et al. Malnutrition associated with unfavorable outcome and death among South African MDR-TB and HIV co-infected children. The international journal of tuberculosis and lung disease : the official journal of the International Union against Tuberculosis and Lung Disease. 2014;18:1074–83.

13. Podewils LJ, Holtz T, Riekstina V, et al. Impact of malnutrition on clinical presentation, clinical course, and mortality in MDR-TB patients. Epidemiology and infection. 2011;139:113–20.

14. Meressa D, Hurtado RM, Andrews JR, et al. Achieving high treatment

success for multidrug-resistant TB in Africa: initiation and scale-up of MDR TB care in Ethiopia--an observational cohort study. Thorax. 2015;70:1181–8.

15. World Health Organization (WHO). WHO treatment guidelines for drug resistant tuberculosis (2016 update) (WHO/HTM/TB/2016.04). Geneva, Switzerland; 2016.

16. Word Health Organization (WHO). Health in 2015 from Millennium Development Goals (MDG) to Sustainable Development Goals (SDG). Geneva, Switzerland; 2015.

17. World Health Organization (WHO). End TB Strategy (WHO/HTM/TB/2015.19). Geneva, Switzerland; 2015.

What happens to TB patients notified from private sector in rural and urban setting? study from Maharashtra, India

Abstract

Background: India accounts for more than 27 % of the global TB burden and 'missing' cases who remain undiagnosed or inadequately diagnosed in the private sector pose a big problem. The Government of India issued a Gazette requiring TB notification (2012) and since that time private sector notifications have increased. Home visits including screening of households and reporting interim/final treatment outcomes occur for patients notified from the public sector, however, little is known about patients notified from private sector.

Methods: This is a descriptive study conducted in seven districts of Maharashtra, India. TB patients notified by private facilities from Jan-March 2018 were interviewed three months after notification by trained staff using a standard and end of treatment outcomes were tracked. Analysis of data was performed using Microsoft Excel.

Results: Of 395 TB patients notified by the private sector, 268 (68%) were males and 353 (89%) had pulmonary TB. Chest radiograph was used in 340 (86%) patients, 45 (11%) underwent smear microscopy, 4 (1%) histopathology, 3 (1 %) USG and 3 (1%) Xpert MTB/RIF assay. Levofloxacin, Ethionamide, Ofloxacin were commonly prescribed with first line anti-TB drugs. Only 79 (20%) people had a home visit by programme staff. At end of treatment, 228 (58%) completed treatment,7 (2%) cured, 6 (2%) died, 1 (0.25%) failed, 51 (13%) lost to follow up, 12 (3 %) transferred out, 2 (1 %) misdiagnosed (cancer/no TB), 19 (5%) changed to public, 39 (10 %) still on private treatment, 30 (8 %) data was not available.

Conclusion: Unfavourable treatment outcomes were high. Quality diagnosis with microbiological confirmation, appropriate treatment and ongoing monitoring is lacking in the private sector. Better linkages between the public and private sector are required to ensure relapse free treatment for private sector.

BACKGROUND

TB is a major public health problem in India accounting to more than 25% of TB burden globally.[1] In India, the country with the largest burden of TB disease, there was a marked increase in both the TB- specific budget and the domestic funding for this budget in 2017. This increase followed high-level (Prime Ministerial) political commitment to an ambitious goal of ending TB by 2025, and the development of a new national strategic plan for TB 2017–2025 that aims to accelerate progress towards this goal.[2] Despite significant gains made by India's revised National TB control programme (RNTCP) in terms of lives saved, India in 2015 and 2016 accounted for one-third and one-fourth of 'missing' 4.3 million patients with TB globally. [1,3]

Most of these 'missing' cases remain undiagnosed or inadequately and unaccountably diagnosed and treated in the private sector.[2] Among TB patients taking outpatient and inpatient care for TB in 2004 in a nationally representative sample, 53% and 44% sought care from private sector respectively.[4] These patients were not reported to national surveillance system. Therefore in 2012, a national policy of mandatory notification and web-based and case-based reporting system (called "Nikshay") was rolled out that facilitated reporting of detected cases by care providers in the public and private sectors (all care providers were engaged through public-public and public-private mix intervention for case finding). [1]

The increase in global TB estimates since 2013 is mostly explained by a continuous increase in notifications in India (+ 37 % between 2013 and 2016). In areas where monitoring was in place, the contribution of PPM to total notifications increased by more than 10% between 2012 and 2016. [1]

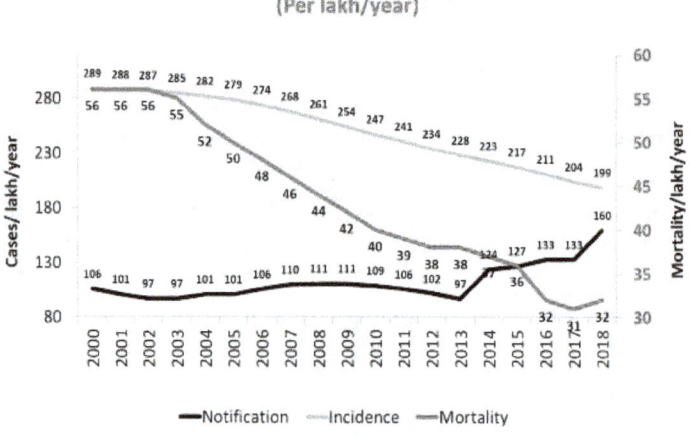

India- Trend in Rate of TB Incidence, Mortality and Notification (Per lakh/year)

Further the below table shows the continous imporvement in TB notification (fig in lakh) in India includding private sector 10-14

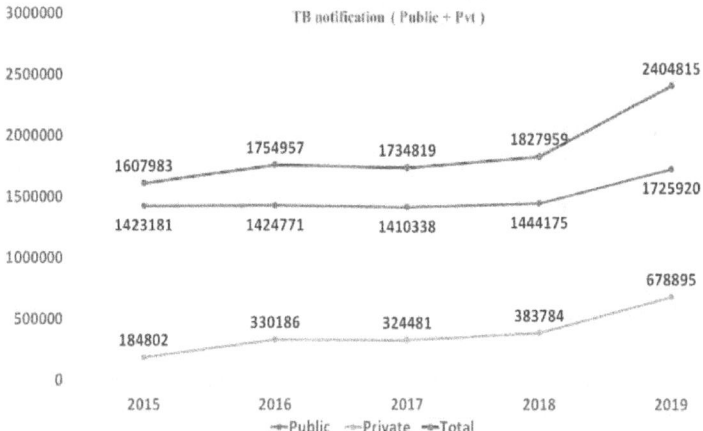

TB notification (Public + Pvt)

Reporting for the interim and final treatment outcomes of patients that are registered for treatment in public facilities and notified under programme settings is in place. However, little is known about what happens to patients notified from private sector: whether they return to Government facility for treatment or take treatment in private sector or are lost to follow up before treatment initiation. Their treatment outcomes are also not routinely reported and tracked. [5] Hence, it is important for the programme to know what happens post-notification to patients notified from the private sector.

AIM AND OBJECTIVES

Among patients with TB (drug susceptible) notified by the private sector during Oct-Dec 2017 (quarter 4) in select six districts of Maharashtra state, India, to describe their characteristics, status after 3 months of notification , public health action initiated by the programme and treatment outcomes at the end of one year/treatment. *Specific objectives* are to determine the:
1. socio-demographic, programmatic and clinical characteristics
2. number (proportion) initiated on treatment in public facility, on treatment in private facility, not on treatment, died at 3 months post-notification.

3. number (proportion) for whom public health action (visit by a programme staff and household contact screening) was initiated by the programme (among those with sputum smear positive TB)
4. treatment outcomes at the end of one year

METHODS

Study design : This is an observational cohort study involving record review.

Settings : Study districts are Aurangabad (Rural) [called as , Aurangabad - MH), Aurangabad municipal corporation, Jalna, Parbhani, Hingoli , Nanded (rural), Nanded (urban) [called as Nanded Waghela MC] of (RNTCP districts) Maharashtra state, India. Following Maharashtra state map depicts the districts highlighted included in study

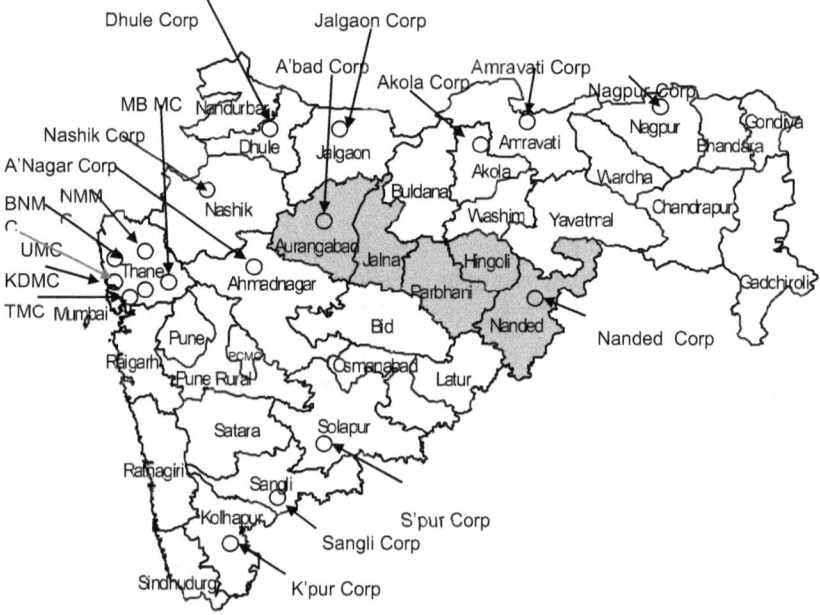

General setting

Maharashtra is the third largest state and is located in western and central India with a population of 119.3 million.[5]. RNTCP infrastructure includes a District TB center for each district (rural) and City TB center for each district (urban) / municipal corporation, sub-district level programme management units called TB units (TUs – one for 500 000 population) and designated microscopic centers

(DMCs – one for 100 000 population) for sputum microscopy. These work under the administrative control of the State TB officer. Patients with presumptive TB visit the DMCs for sputum examination and once diagnosed with TB, the patient is registered at the public health institution (PHI) level for treatment followed by notification to NIKSHAY and entry in TB notification register kept at each PHI. Patient is then allotted a NIKSHAY ID (unique identifier for TB patient under the programme).[6] Laboratory registers maintained in each DMC contain details of each person who underwent sputum smear microscopy and TB notification registers maintained at each PHI indicate the number of TB patients treated under RNTCP. RNTCP has its own quarterly reporting system which is first generated at TU (sub-district administrative unit) level, and then collated at district followed by at state level [7].

TB notification

NIKSHAY is a web enabled and case based monitoring application that has been developed by National Informatics Centre (NIC). Patients registered for treatment at the PHI level and those diagnosed/managed in private sector are notified in NIKSHAY.[8] The TB notification rate for Maharashtra state (159 per lac population) is higher than the national rate of 138 per lac population. In 2017, a total of 192458 patients with TB were notified, of which 67558 (35 %) were notified from the private sector. This is higher than the national figure of 21 % being notified from the private sector. [5]

The population and notification related information of study districts is depicted in **Table 1.** TB notification as a proportion of total notification varies across the districts: as high as 72% in Nanded (urban) and as low as 12% and 18 % in Nanded (rural) and Aurangabad (rural) respectively. [5]

Table 1. Population and notification related details in the select 7 RNTCP districts (study districts) of Maharashtra state, India (2018) [5]

Sr No.	RNTCP district name	Populatio n (in lac)	Total notified (Public)	TB notificatio n rate /L/Y(Public)	Total notifie d (Pvt)	TB notificatio n rate /L/Y(Pvt)	Total TB Notificatio n (G+P)	Notifie d from private sector (%)
1	Aurangaba d MC	12.56	1191	95	649	52	147	35%
2	Aurangaba d (Rural)	26.46	1905	72	413	16	88	18%
3	Jalna	21.26	1508	71	605	28	99	29%
4	Parbhani	19.92	1521	76	400	20	96	21%
5	Hingoli	12.80	876	68	256	20	88	23%
6	Nanded (Rural)	30.45	2853	94	394	13	107	12%

7	Nanded (Urban)	5.74	383	67	998	174	241	72%
	MH	1213.0	124900	103	67558	56	159	35%
	India	13215.0	1444175	109	383784	29	138	21%

Nanded (urban) is notled as Namded Waghala MC, Aurangabad (Rural) is also called as Aurangabad-MH

Follow up of notified patients:

Patients notified from private sector are either form private laboratories or from private health care providers. Their details are routinely filled in the notification register: one for patients notified form private laboratory (annexure I) and one for patients notified from private health care providers (annexure II). The same is maintained as a soft copy (single entry) in MS Excel format. This is done by TB-health visitor and senior treatment supervisor. The details filled here include demographic, clinical and programmatic characteristics (details in annexure I and II shared with this protocol) from notification to follow up examination to treatment outcomes including public health action initiated.

Patient will be tracked for treatment outcomes after 6 months to 1 year of treatment initiation. The programme staff will actively monitor their treatment outcomes and classify them as per the national guidelines which are based on WHO recommendations. [9] **(Table 3)**

Table 3. Treatment outcomes at the end of treatment as per programme guidelines in India which are in line with WHO recommendations [9]

Treatment outcome	Definition
Cured	Completes treatment and is sputum negative at end of treatment.
Treatment completed	Completes treatment but sputum status at the end of treatment not known.
Loss to follow up	Patient does not take ATT for two months continuously due to any reason.
Died	Patient who dies during TB treatment.
Changed to DR-TB regimen	Patient is shifted to DR-TB regimen after being initiated on TB treatment
Failure	Sputum positive at end of 5 months or later
Still on treatment	Continuing treatment as per private practitioner assessment
Not evaluated	Patient whose treatment outcomes are not available (including patient transferred for treatment to other

	private practitioner and the outcomes are not available)
Favourable treatment outcome	Cured, treatment completed
Unfavourable treatment outcome	Loss to follow up, died, change to DR-TB regiment, failure, not evaluated

This is routinely done by the programme staff by contacting the patient and private care provider from time to time.

Study population

All patients with TB notified from the private sector in the study districts during quarter 1st of 2018 (Jan-March 2018) will be included in the study. The estimated sample size is around 900 patients. **(Table 2)**

Table 2. Estimated sample size of the study population in the study

Sr No.	RNTCP district name	Private sector notification in 2017	Estimated notification per quarter in 2018
1	Aurangabad MC	649	162
2	Aurangabad (Rural)	413	103
3	Jalna	605	151
4	Parbhani	400	100
5	Hingoli	256	64
6	Nanded (Rural)	394	99
7	Nanded (Urban)	998	250
	Total		929

Assuming the notification in 2018 is the same as in 2017

Data collection: variables and sources of data:

During 2018, data collection and entry (annexure I and II as described in setting) will done as a part of routine programme activity by programme staff like Senior Treatment Supervisor (STS) and Public Private Mix Coordinator (PPM). Both the staff were trained in data collection by using the standard format used for TB notification from private doctors.

The following variables will be used

Patient unique Id (Nikshay ID)

Date of TB notification

District name:

TU name:

Private health facility name:

Private Health facility type:

Source of notification (Laboratory/single private practitioner clinic/private hospital/others):

Source of notification (specify if mentioned as others above):

Name of PHI under which the private health facility is located

Location of PHI (Urban/rural)

Age in complete yrs

Gender (Male/female/other)

Date of TB diagnosis

Date of initiation of treatment

Status at the time of notification (diagnosed and not initiated on treatment, initiated on treatment, completed treatment)

Type of treatment (Daily) –

New : (Cat I) – Drugs : IP (INH+ETB+RCIN+PZA) + CP (HRE) = 6 months or more

Retreatment (Cat II)- Drugs : IP (INH+ETB+RCIN+PZA+ SM) + CP (HRE) = 8 months or more

Type of TB: pulmonary / extra pulmonary

If extra-pulmonary, which site (LN, pleurisy, abdominal, CNS, renal, others)

Sputum smear status at diagnosis: negative, scanty positive, 1+ positive, 2+ positive, 3+positive, positive not quantified, missing

Culture status at diagnosis if culture done (positive/negative):

HIV status at diagnosis

Weight at diagnosis

DM status at diagnosis

TB treatment outcome (Cured/treatment completed/dead/loss to follow up/ treatment failure/still on treatment / not evaluated/treatment less than one month)

Date of treatment outcome

Data management and analysis:

Data entered (Annexure I and II) in MS Excel will be verified for duplicates and a final list will of study participants will be made. Name, age and sex will be used to identify duplicates. The NIKSHAY identifier provided by the programme will be the unique identifier for the patient. Final line list of dataset after cleaning (Excel sheet) will be imported and analysed using Epi-Data (2.2.2.183 for analysis, EpiData association, Odense, Denmark).

Baseline characteristics of the study population will be summarized in the form of frequency, proportions, mean (SD) and median (IQR). Time intervals between diagnoses, notification, treatment (not always in the same order) will be calculated and summarized in median (IQR) days. The status of patients at 3 months after notification and the treatment outcomes will be compared across subgroups using chi square tests. Levels of significance will be set at 5%.

Results: Below table-1 show distribution of patients according to the variables

Total -1 (n = 465)		
Total patients Notified (1q19) from all study districts	465	%
Number removed from analysis because of discrepant information	70	15%
Total	395	85%

Distribution of cases as per gender (n = 395)		
Male	268	68%
Female	127	32%

Distribution of cases as per type of TB (n = 395)		
Pulmonary	353	89%
Extrapulmonary	42	11%
	395	100 %

Distribution of patients as per the technology used for diagnosis (n = 395)		
Smear microscopy (all pulmonary + 4 EP (microscopy on EP sample)	45	11%
Clinical + X-ray chest	340	86%
CBNAAT /PCR (ALL Pul)	3	1%
Histopathology (EP)	4	1%
USG (EP)	3	1%
Total	395	

Status at three month of treatment (n= 395)		

No specific information available	24	6%
Continue Pvt treatment	294	74%
Shifted to Govt	45	11%
LOST TO FOLLOW UP	24	6%
Not on Treatment	6	2%
Died	1	0%
Pts not on address	1	0%
	395	100%

Status at the end of treatment (n= 395)

No specific information available	29	7%
Still on Pvt treatment	39	10%
Changed to public treatment	19	5%
TC	228	58%
Cured	7	2%
Died	6	2%
Failure	1	0.3%
Misdiagnosed (1 - cancer; 1- no TB)	2	1%
Admitted in edical college	1	0.3%
Lost to F/U	51	13%
TO	12	3%
Total	308	100

Distribution of cases as per home visit and counselling by staff (n = 395)

Home visit done	79	20%
STS	54	68%
TBHV	2	3%
MPW	12	15%
PPM	11	14%
Home visit not done	316	80%

Age sex wise distribution (n=395)			
Age group	Total (n)	Male	Female
0-14	14 (4%)	8 (57 %)	6 (43 %)
15-24	76 (19%)	49 (64 %)	27 (36 %)
25-34	83 (21%)	51 (61 %)	32 (39 %)
35-44	67 (17 %)	48 (72 %)	19 (28 %)
45-54	70 (18%)	49 (70 %)	21 **(30 %)**
55-64	55 (14%)	39 (71 %)	16 (29 %)
65-74	21 (5%)	17 (81	4 (19 %)
75-84	8 (2%)	6 (75 %)	2 (25 %)
85 +	1 (0.3%)	1 (100 %)	0
	395	268 (68)	127 (32)

Of 395 TB patients notified by the private sector, 268 (68%) were males and 353 (89%) had pulmonary TB. Chest radiograph was used in 340 (86%) patients, 45 (11%) underwent smear microscopy, 4 (1%) histopathology, 3 (1 %) USG and 3 (1%) Xpert MTB/RIF assay.

Levofloxacin, Ethionamide, Ofloxacin were commonly prescribed with first line anti-TB drugs.

Only 79 (20%) people had a home visit by programme staff. At end of treatment, 228 (58%) completed treatment, 7 (2%) cured, 6 (2%) died, 1 (0.25%) failed, 51 (13%) lost to follow up, 12 (3 %) transferred out, 2 (1 %) misdiagnosed (cancer/no TB), 19 (5%) changed to public, 39 (10 %) still on private treatment, 30 (8 %) data was not available.

Conclusion:

Unfavourable treatment outcomes were high. Quality diagnosis with microbiological confirmation, appropriate treatment and ongoing monitoring is lacking in the private sector. Better linkages between the public and private sector are required to ensure relapse free treatment for private sector.

Ethics approval

Ethics Issues: Permission for the study has been sought from TB programme manager (Joint Director of Health Services), Government of Maharashtra. Ethics approval will be sought from the Union Ethics Advisory Group, Paris, France. The PI does not have access to a local ethics committee. As this study, involves review of existing records (secondary data) within the programme we request a waiver for informed consent.

Data confidentiality: Annexure I and II are records within the programme. The final dataset in Excel format will be kept in a password protected computers accessible only to the investigators.

Specific patient benefits: There will not be direct patient benefits. The results of this study will inform the programme about status of patients with TB that are notified to the programme from the private sector. This may result in better management of such patient in future.

Community participation and benefits: There are no direct benefits. These are likely to arise from the study in that status and outcomes of TB patients notified by private providers will be available with the programme The results can help in evidence based advocacy for TB notification among the stakeholders.

Feedback and dissemination of results: The results of this study will be disseminated to programme managers, health care workers in the NTP, patient care groups and the private health care providers in the study districts. The results will also be presented at national and international conferences and submitted in a peer reviewed journal.

Implications for policy and practice: There may be implications for policy and practice depending on results of the study. If the results indicate that the outcomes are poor and majority are not traceable post notification, then this will act as an advocacy tools for these patients to be linked to care under programme. If outcomes are good, the existing model of care would be continued.

Collaborative partnerships: these will be between the WHO country office in India, Health services of Government of Maharashtra, South East Asia Office of The Union, New Delhi.

REFERENCES

1. World Health Organization (WHO). Global tuberculosis report 2017. WHO/HTM/TB/2017.23. Geneva, Switzerland; 2017.
2. Revised National Tuberculosis Control Programme (RNTCP); Central TB Division. National strategic plan for TB elimination 2017-25. New Delhi, India; 2017.
3. World Health Organization (WHO). Global Tuberculosis Report 2016. Geneva, Switzerland; 2016.
4. Hazarika I. Role of private sector in providing tuberculosis care: Evidence from a population-based survey in India. J Glob Infect Dis. 2011;3(1):19.
5. Revised National Tuberculosis Control Programme (RNTCP). TB India

2018. Annual status report. New Delhi India; 2018.

6. Revised National Tuberculosis Control Programme (RNTCP) Central TB Division. Diagnosis of smear positive pulmonary TB. New Delhi India; 2009.

7. Revised National Tuberculosis Control Programme (RNTCP). Central TB Division. Ministry of Health and Family Welfare. Government of India. Technical and operational guidelines for tuberculosis control in India. New Delhi India; 2016.

8. Revised national tuberculosis control programme (RNTCP); Central TB division; Ministry of Health and Family Welfare; Government of India. NISHAY - A web based solution for monitoring of TB patients [Internet]. [cited 2017 Nov 15]. Available from: https://nikshay.gov.in/AboutNikshay.htm

9. World Health Organization (WHO). Definitions and Reporting Framework for Tuberculosis- 2013 revision (updated December 2014). Geneva, Switzerland; 2014.

10. India TB Report 2016, , NATIONAL TUBERCULOSIS ELIMINATION PROGRAMME ANNUAL REPORT Central TB Division Ministry of Health and Family Welfare, Nirman Bhawan, New Delhi - 110011 www.tbcindia.gov.in

11. India TB Report 2017, , NATIONAL TUBERCULOSIS ELIMINATION PROGRAMME ANNUAL REPORT Central TB Division Ministry of Health and Family Welfare, Nirman Bhawan, New Delhi - 110011 www.tbcindia.gov.in

12. India TB Report 2018, , NATIONAL TUBERCULOSIS ELIMINATION PROGRAMME ANNUAL REPORT Central TB Division Ministry of Health and Family Welfare, Nirman Bhawan, New Delhi - 110011 www.tbcindia.gov.in

13. India TB Report 2019, , NATIONAL TUBERCULOSIS ELIMINATION PROGRAMME ANNUAL REPORT Central TB Division Ministry of Health and Family Welfare, Nirman Bhawan, New Delhi - 110011 www.tbcindia.gov.in

14. India TB Report 2020, , NATIONAL TUBERCULOSIS ELIMINATION PROGRAMME ANNUAL REPORT Central TB Division Ministry of Health and Family Welfare, Nirman Bhawan, New Delhi - 110011 www.tbcindia.gov.in

ANNEXURES

Annexures for patients notified form private laboratory (annexure I) and one for patients notified from private health care providers (annexure II) have been attached as separate MS Excel files along with this proposal.

TB Notification reporting format for Medical Laboratory

Period of reporting: From ...../...../...... To ...../...../......

Name of the Laboratory :...   Health Establishment code for TB Notification

Registration Number:.............................. Telephone (with STD):..........................   ..../................

Mobile number:............................

Complete Address: ....

Sr. No.	Name of TB Patient (surname first)	Father / Husband's name	Age (yrs)	Sex (M/ F/O)	Gol issued identification number	Complete residential address	PIN number	Patient Phone number	Date of TB Diag-nosis*	Date of sputum collection	Date of result	Type of Test result (smear microscopy positive / culture positive / MTB on LPA / MTB on Xpert / MTB in FNAC / TB on Histopath/ DST	DST results for each drug tested (Rif-resistant / S-sensitive/NA-not available) Rif, INH, SM, EMB, Ofx, Km, Eto, Cipro, Capr. etc.						
													Rif	INH	SM	EMB	Ofx	Km	

* Mandatory

Laboratories include those Health Establishments carrying out any of the RNTCP endorsed TB diagnostics

Signature:..   Date: ...../...../......

Annexure II   **TB Notification reporting format for**
Medical practitioners/Clinics/Hospitals/Nursing homes

Period of reporting: From ...../...../...... To ...../...../......

Name of the health facility / practitioner :...(single/Multi) Health Establishment code for TB Notification

Registration Number:.. Telephone (with STD):...........................   ..../................

Mobile number:............................

Complete Address: ....

Sr. No.	Name of TB Patient (surname first)	Father / Husband's name	Age (yrs)	Sex (M/ F/O)	Gol issued identification number *	Complete residential address	PIN no.	Patient Phone number	Date of TB Diagnosis *	Date of TB treatment initiation*	Site of Disease (P /EP)*	Patient Type (New TB case/ Recurrent TB case/ Treatment changes) *	Basis of diagnosis (Smear microscopy/ culture / PCR/ LPA/ FNAC/Histo-pathology/Clinical exam/X-Ray)	Weight in Kg.	Drugs and dosages (in mg) H/R/Z/E/S/ Ofx/Cs/Eto/ Levo/Mx/Cpr/ Other (specify)

* Mandatory

Private practitioner / Clinic (single) will include any Health Establishments where TB cases are treated or diagnosed clinically / radiologically and the medical services are provided by single medical practitioner.

Hospital / Clinic / Nursing Home (multi-practitioners) will include any Health Establishments where TB cases are treated or diagnosed clinically/radiologically & medical services are provided by more than one practitioner.

Signature:..   Date: ...../...../......

[PART I—SEC.1] भारत का राजपत्र : असाधारण 13

Annexure II

TB Notification reporting format for
Medical practitioners / Clinics/Hospitals/Nursing homes

Period of reporting: From ...../......./...... To ...../......./.....

Name of the health facility / practitioner :...(single/Multi)   Health Establishment code for TB Notification

Registration Number:...................................... Telephone (with STD):...........................   ..../...........
Mobile number:...............................
Complete Address: ....

Pa-tient ID	Pa-tient home visit Done (Y/N)	If Yes, done by	Pa-tient coun-seling Done (Y/N)	Type of treat-ment adher-ence (DOT/ SMS/ Phone/99 DOT/Vid eo DOT/Pill box/ SAT)	Status of patient (regu-lar/ Not regu-lar)	Month at which FU examina-tion done	Status at FU exam-ination (SM/Cult) (Pos/Neg)	Clinical improve-ment (Yes/No)	No, of con-tacts	No, of contact symp-tomatic	No, found to have TB among contact	No, of con-tacts initiat-ed on anti-TB treat-ment	No, of contacts offered chem-oprophylaxis	HIV test-ing of-fered (No/Neg/ Pos)	DST offered (No/RIF resistance /RIF sensi-tive/ Indetermi-nate)	Treatment Outcome (C/TC/F/D/ LTFU/TO/ RC)

C=Cured, TC=Treatment Completed F=Failure D=Died LTFU=Lost to Follow Up TO=Transferred Out RC =Regimen Change.
This information on page 2 is to be submitted during treatment and after treatment completion with sos updation in Nikshay with public health action support by local public health staff.
Signature:...   Date : ...../......./......

35

Publisher: Eliva Press SRL

Email: info@elivapress.com

Eliva Press is an independent publishing house established for the publication and dissemination of academic works all over the world. Company provides high quality and professional service for all of our authors.

Our Services:
Free of charge, open-minded, eco-friendly, innovational.

-All services are free of charge for you as our author (manuscript review, step-by-step book preparation, publication, distribution, and marketing).
-No financial risk. The author is not obliged to pay any hidden fees for publication.
-Editors. Dedicated editors will assist step by step through the projects.
-Money paid to the author for every book sold. Up to 50% royalties guaranteed.
-ISBN (International Standard Book Number). We assign a unique ISBN to every Eliva Press book.
-Digital archive storage. Books will be available online for a long time. We don't need to have a stock of our titles. No unsold copies. Eliva Press uses environment friendly print on demand technology that limits the needs of publishing business. We care about environment and share these principles with our customers.
-Cover design. Cover art is designed by a professional designer.
-Worldwide distribution. We continue expanding our distribution channels to make sure that all readers have access to our books.

www.elivapress.com

www.ingramcontent.com/pod-product-compliance
Lightning Source LLC
Chambersburg PA
CBHW072045190526
45165CB00018B/1824